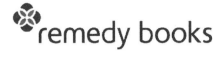

Concepts in Health Care Entrepreneurship
Clinic Checklist

Author: Jenson Hagen, CPA, MSFA

Has worked for some of the top investment and accounting firms in the nation. Has passed six professional examinations in various areas of business, including the Certified Public Accountant exam and Level II of the Chartered Financial Analyst exam. Holds an M.S. degree in Financial Analysis, a program of study that provides detailed training on how to conduct business valuations.

Contributing Author: John M. Hagen, DC

Runs a highly successful practice in the Vancouver, Washington area. Has over 30 years of experience as a doctor of chiropractic. Developed many of the concepts related to patient care.

Copyright @ 2012 Remedy Books

PO Box 1182
Portland, OR 97207

Library of Congress Control Number: 2012922350

ISBN: 978-0-9839510-2-5

For permission to use material from this clinic checklist, please submit a request using our online submission form at remedybooks.com or email info@remedybooks.com

Peer review provided by Amanda Buffington.

Warning: This book has not been technically reviewed for accuracy.

The publisher or copyright owner is not responsible as a matter of liability, negligence, or otherwise for any injury resulting from any material contained in this book. Concepts described in this book have not been technically reviewed for accuracy and could contain errors or misstatements. This clinic checklist does not cover all of the items a person may need to start and operate a health care clinic and should not be solely relied upon when making business decisions.

Table of Contents

This clinic checklist provides important detail to consider when starting a new health care organization, developing one, or simply trying to make modifications. This checklist is best read in tandem with our textbook, Concepts in Health Care Entrepreneurship, which you can find online at remedybooks.com.

Not every item on this list is important for your success. You must gauge the nature of your own organization and financial situation to determine what items to consider. Keep note of what vendor offers the best price related to each particular item. You may want to purchase products or services from a vendor within your community to support referrals and word of mouth even if the price is not the best. Use a pencil when filling out this checklist in order to modify the vendor, price, or expected quantity at a later moment.

Put together a growth plan to develop your clinic in stages. Be careful not to grow beyond your management abilities or financial means. Use the columns labeled 1 2 3 to establish three stages of a growth plan and identify the stage in which a particular item will be purchased. Again, not every item mentioned in this checklist will be applicable to your organization.

Use the notes section on the back of each page to keep track of additional information not covered by the checklist. Maintaining good notes will prove helpful if significant time passes between identifying an item during the planning of your clinic and performing a task or making a purchase later. The notes section can also be used to provide more detail on your growth plan.

Please review the free resources found online at remedybooks.com. Amounts compiled on the checklist can be tabulated and placed on the budgets and ratios spreadsheet found under the *Students* tab.

Goal Boards

Placement areas

Breakroom ☐

Home ☐

Journal notebook ☐

Office ☐

Contents

Goals ☐

Action steps ☐

Key success factors ☐

Metrics ☐

Balanced Scorecard[1]

Financial perspective

Debt levels ☐

Net profit ☐

Revenue ☐

Savings ☐

Internal processes perspective

Administrative procedures ☐

Communication systems ☐

Information technology ☐

Job duties ☐

Learning and growth perspective

Asset purchases ☐

Business plan ☐

Continuing education ☐

Training ☐

Patient perspective

Feedback ☐

Health care procedures ☐

Retention analysis ☐

Surveys ☐

Growth Plan

Metrics specify when to move to the next stage of a growth plan.

Employee pay or benefits ☐

Hire new employees or contractors ☐

Modify job duties ☐

Relocate or renovate ☐

Equipment purchases ☐

Marketing campaigns ☐

Offer new products or services ☐

Upgrade information technology ☐

Succession Plan

Specify the process to follow if a business partner, key employee, or you leave or pass away.

Business partner liabilities ☐

Communication system ☐

Professional assistance (attorney, CPA) ☐

Sale of patient base (list potential buyers) ☐

Family obligations (buy out surviving spouse) ☐

Partnership agreement terms and conditions ☐

Replacements (employee, alternate provider) ☐

Sale of property (list potential buyers) ☐

Transition Options

Consider ways to transition from school into your own clinic.

Buy a large practice at once or in stages ☐

Buy a small practice to increase your patient base ☐

Form a new clinic alone or in partnership ☐

Share space and control your own profit ☐

Work as an associate but retain patients ☐

Work for and then buy a franchise office ☐

Work part time and grow a patient base ☐

Work full time and save money ☐

[1] The balanced scorecard is a management device used to organize goals created by Drs Robert Kaplan and David Norton.

Notes

Macroeconomic Outlook

Speak with an SBA or SCORE office to gather information.

Business cycle (current stage) _____   Business cycle (future stage in 3-5 years) _____

Conference Board Leading Economic Index™ _____   Estimated inflation rate (next 3-5 years) _____

Industry cycle (current stage) _____   Industry cycle (future stage in 3-5 years) _____

Website list

Bloomberg News	bloomberg.com	Financial news
Bureau of Economic Analysis	bea.gov	U.S. GDP and balance of trade
Bureau of Labor Statistics	bls.gov	U.S. employment and inflation
Daily FX	dailyfx.com/calendar	Global economic calendar
Economic Indicators	economicindicators.gov	U.S. leading economic indicators
Federal Reserve Bank of NY	ny.frb.org	U.S. central bank
Reuters	reuters.com	Business and financial news

Microeconomic Outlook

Read newspapers and speak with your state's licensing board and professional association to gather information.

Consumer trends _____

_____

Health care trends _____

_____

Legislative activity _____

_____

Competitor Analysis

Meet with other health care providers in your marketplace and ask if they are satisfied with profit levels.

Competitors/Substitutes	Products and services	Price range	Hours	Satisfied?
_____	_____	_____	_____	_____
_____	_____	_____	_____	_____
_____	_____	_____	_____	_____
_____	_____	_____	_____	_____
_____	_____	_____	_____	_____
_____	_____	_____	_____	_____
_____	_____	_____	_____	_____

How will your organization react to competitive pressures?

New skills or services _____

New target markets _____

Notes

Competitor Analysis

Questions to ask when meeting with competitors, including ones that offer substitute products and services.

Do your profit levels meet expectations? ☐
Do you have any plans to increase price levels? ☐
Do you allow patients to set special appointments? ☐
Do you feel that competitive pressures are high? ☐
Have any marketing efforts (not) worked for you? ☐
Would you recommend focusing on any target market? ☐
Would you recommend any professionals to obtain services from? ☐

Marketplace

Item	Vendor	Price	No	Total
Map				
Markers				
Pins				

Draw out marketing zones ☐   Pin target items ☐

Contact the city planning office and drive around your area to better understand your marketplace.

Development projects _____

Growth potential _____

Transportation options _____

Unemployment _____

Unused land _____

Organization

Download the budgets and ratios analysis pack at remedybooks.com under the Students tab to review your clinic.

Breakeven point	☐	Cash budget	☐
Contribution margin	☐	Financial budget	☐
Financial ratios	☐	Marketing analysis	☐
Patient ratios	☐	Operating budget	☐
Sensitivity analysis	☐	SWOT analysis	☐

Service Mix

List the services you plan to offer.

Service line	Price	Special equipment	Target market

Notes

Territory Management

People

List everyone that could help with marketing efforts. Use customer relationship management (CRM) software to organize your territory or download a territory worksheet at remedybook.com under the Students tab.

Acquaintances		Business owners	
Classmates		Coworkers	
Employees (your own)		Employees (other businesses)	
Family		Friends	
Neighbors		Professionals	
Referral sources (current)		Target markets	

Target Markets

Community organizations		Demographic variables	
Geographic locations		Interests and hobbies	
Occupations		Specific health conditions	

Website list

Google Contacts	google.com/contacts	Integrates with Gmail
Daylite by Marketcircle	marketcircle.com	CRM program for Apple
Outlook 2010 with Business Contact Manager	microsoft.com	CRM program
Prophet 5	avidian.com	Integrates with Outlook
Sage Act!	act.com	CRM program

Places

Apartment complexes		Banks	
Coffee shops		Community centers	
Convention centers (hotels)		Grocery stores	
Gyms		Health food stores	
Insurance brokers		Law firms	
Local neighborhoods		Parks	
Places of worship		Restaurants	
Shopping malls		Strip malls	
Theatres		Yoga studios	

Events

BBQs		Charity	
Community talks		Community events (general)	
Concerts		Conventions	
Festivals		Fundraising	
Open house		Parades	
Picnics		Radio shows	
Religious		Sales luncheons	
Seminars		Sports	

Notes

Marketing Tools

Advertisements

Billboards	☐	Busses	☐
Flyer boards	☐	Journals	☐
Magazines	☐	Menus	☐
Newsletters	☐	Newspapers	☐
Personal assets (car)	☐	Restaurants	☐

Collateral

Items can be created using an office suite or graphic designer.

Item	Vendor	Price	No	Total	1	2	3
Brochures (about clinic)							
Brochures (health)							
Business cards							
Direct mailers							
Flyers							
Holiday cards							
Letterhead							
Logo							
Newsletters							
Reminder cards							
Thank you cards							

Media Spots

Item	Producer	Price	No	Total	1	2	3
Radio							
TV							
Video							
Webinar							

Websites

Domain name registration and webserver hosting is often offered with blog and all-in-one services. Title tags are what search engines use to rank your website in search results.

All-in-one service (weebly.com, wordpress.com)	☐	Blog (blogger.com)	☐
Bookmark useful websites	☐	Put in <title> title tag references </title>	☐

Item	Vendor	Total	1	2	3
Appointment manager (schedulicity.com)					
Register domain name (godaddy.com)					
Template (modify in Dreamweaver)					
Webserver (godaddy.com)					

Total for page _____

15

Notes

Marketing Tools

Price Incentives

Coupons

No-obligation consultation

Discounts (cash payers)

Value items (upsell customers later)

Promotional Items

Item	Vendor	Price	No	Total	1	2	3
Awareness bracelets							
Bookmarks							
Bumper stickers							
Calendars							
Health care products							
Magnets							
Mugs							
Pens							
Shirts							
Stress balls							

Website list

4imprint	4imprint.com
Branders.com	branders.com
Cintas	cintaspromoproducts.com
Staples	staplespromotionalproducts.com
Zazzle	zazzle.com

Narratives

Prearranged, memorized dialogue to ensure key information is communicated in a clear and professional manner.

Address sales resistance (time, money, energy)

Instructions on how to make a referral or spread word of mouth

Describe products or services

Total for page _____

Notes

Narratives

Describe upcoming events

Describe services or products

Describe your profession

Describe yourself

Highlight your organization

Provide a quality guarantee

Termination of employee

Notes

Collateral Transmission

Item	Vendor	Postage	Total	1	2	3
Advertise in a coupon book	_____	_____	_____			
Mail brochures or cards (thank you, holiday)	_____	_____	_____			

Display business cards with area businesses	☐	Email newsletters	☐
Hand out brochures or flyers (neighborhood)		Hand out business cards	

Community Groups

Charities	☐	Meet-ups	☐
Personal hobbies and interests		Philanthropy	
Political		Public speaking (toastmasters.org)	
Religious		Sports	

Website list

Kiwanis International	kiwanis.org	Focused on children
Lions Club International	lionsclubs.org	Serving the community
National Association of Investors Corp	betterinvesting.org	Investment club
Optimist International	optimist.org	Focused on children
Rotary International	rotary.org	Serving the community
Soroptimist International	soroptimist.org	Women's club
U.S. Chamber of Commerce	uschamber.com	Business federation

Convention Booth

Item	Vendor	Price	No	Total	1	2	3
Banner	_____	_____	_____	_____			
Cardboard cutout	_____	_____	_____	_____			
Folding chair	_____	_____	_____	_____			
Folding table	_____	_____	_____	_____			
Healthy treats	_____	_____	_____	_____			

Brochures	☐	Business cards	☐
Discount coupons		Narratives	
Promotional items		Treatment table	

Gather Feedback

Direct communication	☐	Mail-in surveys	☐
Personal meetings		Questionnaires	
Suggestion box		Survey forms	

Total for page _____

Notes

Hold Classes

Diet	☐	Exercise	☐
General wellbeing	☐	Preventative medicine	☐
Specific health topics	☐	Sports medicine	☐
Supplements	☐	Weight loss	☐

Class venues

Community college (adult course)	☐	Local business	☐
In-house	☐	Online	☐

Online

Item	Vendor	Price	No	Total	1	2	3
Bing Ads	bingads.microsoft.com	_____	____	_____			
Google AdWords	adwords.google.com	_____	____	_____			

Advertise on community member websites	☐	Coupon deals (Groupon, LivingSocial)	☐
Facebook business page and posts	☐	Google Places	☐
LinkedIn profile	☐	Monitor online reviews of your business	☐
Twitter feed	☐	YouTube video	☐

Open House

Item	Vendor	Price	No	Total	1	2	3
Beverages	_____	_____	____	_____			
Food	_____	_____	____	_____			

Brochures	☐	Business cards	☐
Discount coupons	☐	Flyers (advertising event)	☐
Promotional items	☐	Narratives including keynote speech	☐

Sales Luncheon

Work through the sales luncheon project found online at remedybooks.com under the Teachers tab.

Item	Vendor	Price	No	Total	1	2	3
Beverages	_____	_____	____	_____			
Food	_____	_____	____	_____			

Brochures	☐	Business cards	☐
Discount coupons	☐	List of attendees	☐
Narratives including keynote speech	☐	Thank you card	☐

Total for page _____

Notes

Architect

Building and land blueprints	Building code and zoning
Interior layout	Review lease limitations

Name _____   Price quote _____

1	2	3

Attorney

Associate contract (retain your patients)	*At will* or *for cause* employee termination
Business form (S corporation, LLC)	Corporate governance (annual meeting)
Covenant not to compete	Employee handbook
Employment laws (applicable ones)	Loan agreement
Partnership agreement	Review lease terms
Termination of employee	Will and estate planning

Name _____   Price quote _____

1	2	3

Bookkeeper

Bank reconciliation	Chart of accounts
Data entry	Internal controls (cash and vendors)
Journal entries	Payroll processing (consider a payroll service)

Name _____   Price quote _____

1	2	3

Business Coach

Administrative processes	Employee management
General advice	Goal setting
Information systems	Information technology
Insurance billing	Job duties
Market analysis	Marketing support

Name _____   Price quote _____

1	2	3

Commercial Real Estate Agent

Location selection with poper zoning	Negotiation of terms

Name _____   Price quote _____

1	2	3

Total for page _____   25

Notes

Employment Agency

Preregister in case an employee suddenly leaves.

Hiring and interview assistance ☐   Temp-to-hire ☐
Temporary worker (special projects) ☐   Wage and benefit determination

	1	2	3

Name _____   Price quote _____

Financial Advisor

Estate planning ☐   Insurance products ☐
Retirement plan management ☐   Wealth management

	1	2	3

Name _____   Price quote _____

Graphic Designer

Logo ☐   Marketing tools ☐
Office documents ☐   Signage ☐
Templates (paper and electronic) ☐   Website

	1	2	3

Name _____   Price quote _____

Insurance Agent

Auto (employee use) ☐   Business continuity ☐
Health (personal or business policy) ☐   Liability ☐
Life ☐   Malpractice ☐
Property ☐   Worker's compensation (select states)

	1	2	3

Name _____   Price quote _____

Interior Designer

Decorations ☐   Energy and mood enhancement ☐
Furniture ☐   Paint colors

	1	2	3

Name _____   Price quote _____

Total for page _____   27

Notes

Payroll Service

Employee benefit administration ☐ Payroll processing ☐
Payroll tax filings and payment submissions ☐ Retirement plan administration ☐

1	2	3
☐	☐	☐

Name _____ Price quote _____

Website list

ADP	adp.com
Paychex	paychex.com

Small Business Administration and SCORE

Go online to sba.gov and score.org to learn more.

Business classes and mentoring ☐ Business plan assistance ☐
Economic research ☐ Loan application assistance ☐

1	2	3
☐	☐	☐

Name _____ Price quote _____

Support Network

Brainstorm ideas and practice sales techniques. Ask specific members of your support network to review your business using a retention checklist found online at remedybooks.com under the Students tab.

Counselor (career, mental health) ☐ Health care providers (mentor) ☐
Fellow students ☐ Psychologist ☐
Professionals in other fields ☐ Small business owners ☐

1	2	3
☐	☐	☐

Name _____ Price quote _____

Tax Accountant (CPA)

Download an accounting methods overview at remedybooks.com under the Students tab.

Accounting methods (cash or accrual) ☐ Business form (S corporation, LLC) ☐
Bookeeping resources ☐ Capital lease requirements ☐
Chart of accounts ☐ Estimated quarterly tax payments ☐
Estimated tax rate for financial analysis ☐ File business license ☐
File Form 2553 for S corporation status ☐ File Form SS-4, Employer Identification Number ☐
File federal and state tax forms ☐ File payroll forms (consider a payroll service) ☐
Internal controls ☐ Qualified employee benefits (cafeteria plan) ☐
Retirement plan selection ☐ Register business form and name with state ☐
Register employment activity ☐ State and local taxes (applicable ones) ☐
Tax planning (end of year) ☐ Worker status verification ☐

1	2	3
☐	☐	☐

Name _____ Price quote _____

Total for page _____

Notes

Office Renovation

Be aware that amounts spent to renovate leased office space may not be recuperated upon vacating the property.

Internal Construction

Item	Vendor	Material	Labor	Total	1	2	3
Air conditioning system							
Air filtration system							
Carpet (hypoallergenic)							
Ceiling fan							
Demolition							
Doors							
Electric							
Flooring							
Insulaton							
Lighting							
Paint (nontoxic)							
Plumbing							
Woodwork (sustainable)							

External Construction

Item	Vendor	Material	Labor	Total	1	2	3
Asphalt							
Awning							
Fencing							
Landscaping							
Gutters							
Roof							
Sidewalks							
Siding							
Solar panels							
Sprinkler system							
Windows (double pane)							

General Tasks

City inspection ☐ Ecofriendly materials ☐
Gather ideas (pinterest.com, magazines) ☐ Review city zoning and building code ☐

Item	Vendor and costs	Total	1	2	3
City permit					
Interior design magazines					
Rezoning					

Total for page _____

Notes

Landscaping Supplies

Item	Vendor	Price	No	Total	1	2	3
Bark							
Clippers							
Fertilizer							
Hedge trimmer							
Hose							
Hoze nozzle							
Lawn mower							
Mulch							
Plants							
Pots							
Rake							
Shrubs							
Sprinkler							
Stepping stones							
Weedeater							

Outside Supplies

Item	Vendor	Price	No	Total	1	2	3
Deicing salts							
Drill							
Extension cord							
Flashlight							
Floodlight (motion sensor)							
Garbage can							
Hammer							
Insect control							
Ladder							
Lamppost							
Measuring tape							
Mouse trap							
Paint (external siding)							
Paint (parking spots)							
Saw							
Shovel							
Smoking receptacle							
Snow shovel							
Tool set							
Vehicle stop							

Total for page _____

Notes

External Environment

Maintenance

Deice walkways ☐	Mow lawn ☐
Fix potholes ☐	Fix sidewalk cracks ☐
Pick up garbage (neighborhood) ☐	Pull weeds ☐
Rake leaves ☐	Remove debris ☐
Remove hazards ☐	Shovel snow ☐
Sweep walkways ☐	Trim hedges ☐
Wash siding ☐	Wash windows ☐

Neighborhood

Amenities for patients ☐	Cleanliness ☐
Coupons to surrounding businesses ☐	Safety (neighborhood watch) ☐

Security Equipment

Item	Vendor	Price	No	Total	1	2	3
Alarm system							
Deadbolt							
Light timer							
Lock							
Security camera							
Window bars							
Window dowel							

Signage

Item	Vendor	Price	No	Total	1	2	3
Business name							
Disabled parking spot							
Enter							
Exit							
Hours of operation							
Neon display							
Nonsmoking signs							
Open and closed							
Parking							
Safety							
Sandwich board							
Smoking area							
Tow away zone							
Window lettering							

Website list

Fast Signs	fastsigns.com
Vistaprint	vistaprint.com

Total for page _____

Notes

Bathroom

Item	Vendor	Price	No	Total	1	2	3
Air freshener							
Air freshener dispenser							
Air hand dryer							
Candle (battery powered)							
Clog remover							
Disability railing							
Facial tissues							
Floor mat or rug							
Hand lotion							
Hand sanitizer							
Hand sanitizer dispenser							
Light fixture (motion)							
Mirror							
Nightlight							
Paper towels							
Paper towel dispenser							
Plunger							
Soap							
Soap dispenser							
Toilet bowl brush							
Toilet bowl cover							
Toilet bowl freshener							
Toilet bowl mat or rug							
Toilet paper							
Toilet paper holder							
Toilet seat covers							

Entertainment

Item	Vendor	Price	No	Total	1	2	3
Binders (articles, testimonials)							
Books (general interest)							
Books (health, nutrition)							
Cookbooks							
DVD player							
DVDs							
Headphones							
Journals (cut out articles)							
Magazines (cut out articles)							
Music CDs							
Music subscription							
Speakers							
Stereo equipment							
Television							
Testimonials							
Toys (chocking hazard)							
Word games							

Total for page _____

Notes

Floor

Item	Vendor	Price	No	Total	1	2	3
Bookcase (supplements)							
Chair							
Coat rack							
Coffee table							
Door mat							
Floor mat							
Lamp							
Lamp table							
Magazine rack							
Plants							
Pots							
Recliner chair (massage)							
Standing light							
Umbrella holder							
Umbrella							

Front Counter

Present information in other languages depending on your patient base. Display a calendar to help patients schedule their next appointment.

Item	Vendor	Price	No	Total	1	2	3
Basket							
Bowl							
Brochure holder							
Business card holder							
Calendar (for patients)							
Flower vase							
Flowers (hypoallergenic)							
Healthy treats							
Hours of operation							
Pens							
Plant							
Sign-in sheet							

Products for sale

Books	☐	Cookbooks	☐
Community member products (cross-referrals)	☐	Exercise equipment	☐
Health treats	☐	Orthopedic equipment	☐
Pillows	☐	Videos	☐

Total for page _____

Notes

Refreshments

Item	Vendor	Price	No	Total	1	2	3
Bottled water dispenser							
Bottled water jug							
Coffee dispenser							
Cream or milk dispenser							
Cups							
Doyle							
Hot water dispenser							
Juice							
Juice container							
Mugs							
Stevia (sweetener)							
Spoons							
Stirring sticks							
Table or stand							
Table cloth							
Tea bags							
Tray							
Water pitcher (lemon, mint)							

Signs

Item	Vendor	Price	No	Total	1	2	3
Bathroom (door)							
Do not enter (door)							

Biohazard	☐	Call 911 in case of emergency (voicemail greeting)	☐
Caution hot beverages	☐	Change to insurance or contact information	☐
Elevators (in case of fire use staircase)	☐	Exit routes in every room with floorplan	☐
Health department (employees must wash hands)	☐	Payment methods accepted	☐
Supplement quality guarantee	☐	Warning labels (supplements, toys)	☐

Walls

Item	Vendor	Price	No	Total	1	2	3
Accolade							
Chart holder							
Clock							
Coat hook (bathroom)							
Positive quote							
Room numbers							
Paint							
Paint brush							
Paint roller tray							
Picture							
Picture frame							
Plaque							
Poster							

Total for page _____

Notes

Office Expenses

Bank Account

Item	Financial institution	Fees	Total
Box of checks			
Business checking account			
Business payroll account			
Business savings account			

Place limits on check writing (prevent fraud) ☐   Lockbox service ☐

Break Area

Item	Vendor	Price	No	Total	1	2	3
Bowls							
Coffee (decaffeinated)							
Coffee filters							
Coffee maker							
Condiments							
Cream or milk							
Cutlery							
Dishwasher (energy efficient)							
Instant hot water faucet							
Microwave							
Pain relievers							
Plates							
Refrigerator (energy efficient)							
Salt and pepper							
Toaster oven (avoid smells)							

Cleaning Supplies

Item	Vendor	Price	No	Total	1	2	3
Antibacterial wipes							
Bleach							
Broom							
Carpet stain remover							
Clothes hamper							
Dust pan							
Duster							
Garbage bags (ecofriendly)							
Garbage can							
Glass cleaner							
Gloves							
Laundry detergent (gowns)							
Mop							
Mop bucket							
Sponge							
Surface cleaner (nontoxic)							
Toilet bowl cleaner							
Vacuum							

Total for page _____

Notes

Office Equipment

Item	Vendor	Price	No	Total	1	2	3
Air conditioning unit							
Air purifier							
Cell phone							
Copier							
Dehumidifier							
Emergency lights							
Fan							
Fax machine							
Filing cabinet							
Hot water heater							
Office chair							
Phone system							
Printer							
Scanner							
Shredder							
Smoke alarms							
Storage cabinet							
Stool							
Vacuum							
Wall dividers							
Washer and dryer							

Office Supplies

Item	Vendor	Price	No	Total	1	2	3
Address labels							
Adhesive tape							
Air filter screen							
Batteries (rechargeable)							
Binder clips							
Binders							
Blinds							
Calculator							
Calendar (adminstrative)							
Clipboard							
Coarkboard (goal setting)							
Correction tape							
Curtains							
Desk pad							
Doorstop							
Eraser							
File folders							
Floor mat							
Glue							
Headset for phone							
Highlighters							
Hole punch							

Total for page _____   45

Notes

Office Supplies (continued)

Items	Vendor	Price	No	Total	1	2	3
Keys (extra set)							
Label maker							
Large envelopes							
Lightbulbs (full spectrum)							
Mailing envelopes							
Markers							
Notepad							
Packing tape							
Paid stamp							
Paper clip holder							
Paper clips							
Paper tray							
Pen and pencil holder							
Pencils							
Pens							
Postage stamps							
Power cord (surge protection)							
Printer paper							
Received stamp							
Rubber bands							
Ruler							
Scissors							
Shipping boxes							
Shipping tape							
Signature stamp							
Staple remover							
Stapler							
Staples							
Sticky notes							
Storage boxes							
Time stamp							
Toner cartridge							
Uniform							

Website list	
EcoGreenOffice	ecogreenoffice.com
Quill	quill.com
TheGreenOffice	thegreenoffice.com

Safety Equipment

Item	Vendor	Price	No	Total	1	2	3
AED cabinet							
Eyewash station							
Defibrillator (AED)							
Fire blanket							
Fire extinguisher							
First aid kit							
IV mixing station							

Total for page _____

Notes

Office Expenses

Security Equipment

Item	Vendor	Price	No	Total	1	2	3
Door chime (front door)							
Lockbox (petty cash)							
Safe (computer backup)							

Services

Item	Vendor	Price	No	Total	1	2	3
Biohazard container pickup							
Carpet cleaning							
Data backup and storage							
Document shredding							
Interpreters (phone)							
IT support							
Janitorial							
Landscaping							
Laundry							
Live phone messaging							
Medical billing							
Mystery shopper							
Online fax							
Pressure washing							
Security patrol							
Snow plow							
Storage unit							
Upholstery cleaning							
Window washing							
Yard maintenance							

Utilities

Item	Vendor	Price	No	Total	1	2	3
Call forwarding							
Call waiting							
Electricity							
Internet							
Gas							
Garbage							
Phone line							
Recycling							
Sewage							
Voice messaging							
Water							

Total for page _____

Notes

Computer System

Hardware

Item	Vendor	Price	No	Total	1	2	3
Adjustable foot rest							
Backup device							
Blank CDs							
Charge card reader							
Desktop computer							
Document stand							
Ergonomic keyboard							
Ergonomic keyboard pad							
Ergonomic mouse							
Ergonomic mouse pad							
External hard drive							
Flash drive							
Laptop carrying case							
Laptop computer							
Random access memory (RAM)							
Server							
Tablet							
Wireless router							

Software

Item	Vendor	Price	No	Total	1	2	3
Administrative calendar							
Charting							
Charge card processing							
CRM (territory management)							
Electronic health records (EHR)							
Firewall							
Inventory (Quickbooks)							
Office suite (Word, Excel)							
Point of sale							
Practice management							
Quickbooks							
Scheduling							
Virus protection							
Website blocker							

Website list

Office Ally	officeally.com	Office Ally
Practice Fusion	practicefusion.com	Practice Fusion
Eclipse	galactek.com	Galactek Corp
Lytec	lytec.com	McKesson
MacPractice	macpractice.com	MacPractice
NaturaeSoft	naturaesoft.com	NaturaeSoft
Vitera Integrity	viterahealthcare.com	Vitera Healthcare Solutions

Total for page _____

Notes

Medical Equipment

Item	Vendor	Price	No	Total	1	2	3
Audiometer							
Autoclave							
Autorefractor							
Blood pressure monitor							
Bone densitometer							
Colposcope							
Curette							
Dermatoscope							
Dynamometer							
Earwash system							
Electrocardiograph							
Fetal monitor							
Glucometer							
Goniometer							
Hemostat							
Holster monitor							
Holster monitor electrodes							
Humidifier							
Hydrocollator							
Inclinometer							
Infant scale							
Laryngoscope							
Microscope							
Nebulizer							
Opthalmascope							
Otoscope							
Overhead lamp							
Oxygen tank							
Pulse oximeter							
Refrigerator (lab specimens)							
Retinoscope							
Rhinoscope							
Scale with height rod							
Sphygmomanometer							
Spirometer							
Stethoscope							
Tonometer							
Transilluminator							
Tympanometer							
X-ray machine							
X-ray viewer							
Ultrasound							
Ultraviolet lamp							
Vital sign monitor							
Vital sign monitor stand							

Total for page _____

Notes

Medical Supplies

Item	Vendor	Price	No	Total	1	2	3
Alphabet tabs (file folders)							
Analgesic (NSAID)							
Anesthesia (lidocaine)							
Antiseptic (iodine, alcohol)							
Athletic tape							
Bandage wrap							
Bandages							
Biohazard container							
Biopsy punch							
Blood draw tubes							
Blood pressure cuff							
Bolster							
Butterfly needles							
Cotton balls							
Cotton swabs							
Crutches							
Digital camera (derm)							
Electrode pads							
Epinephrine							
Eye chart							
Eye dropper							
Face mask							
File folders (patient charts)							
Forceps							
Gauze pads							
Gowns							
Halogen lights							
Hemostat							
Hot packs							
Ice packs							
Insufflation bulb							
Lab coat							
Liquid nitrogen							
Medical gloves							
Microscope slides							
Needles							
Otoscope covers							
Pen light							
Percussion hammer							
Pinwheel							
Poster (exercise, stretching)							
Power handle							
Safety goggles							
Scalpel							
Sheets							
Specula							
Surgical gloves							
Surgical tray							

Total for page _____

Notes

Medical Supplies (continued)

Item	Vendor	Price	No	Total	1	2	3
Suture material							
Syringe							
Table paper							
Tongue depressor							
Tourniquet							
Tuning fork							
Tweezer							
Two-point discriminator							
Voice recorder							
Wedge block							
Wheelchair							
X-ray film							

Lab Kits

Item	Lab company
Allergy	
Fingerstick glucose	
Fertility and ovulation	
GI health panel	
H. pylori breath test	
Hemoglobin A1C	
HIV antibodies	
Hormone (salivary)	
Lactose or fructose absorption	
Lyme's disease	
Monospot blood test	
Pregnancy	
Rapid strep	
SIBO or lactulose breath test	
TB Mantoux skin test	
Toxic metals	
Urinary dipsticks	
Wet prep	

Research Supplies

Item	Vendor	Price	No	Total	1	2	3
Coding books (ICD)							
Journals							
Magazines							
Manuals (Merck)							
Medical dictionary							
Research database (PubMed)							
Textbooks							

Total for page _____

Notes

Dental Equipment

Item	Vendor	Price	No	Total	1	2	3
Acrylic							
Bonding agent							
Broach							
Burnisher							
Bur							
Caliper							
Cart (all-purpose)							
Carver							
Cement							
Chisel							
Condenser							
Curette							
Dental chair							
Desensitizer							
Drill							
Elevator							
Explorer							
Floss							
Forcep							
Handpiece							
Hatchet							
Mouth mirror							
Mouth rinse (fluoridated)							
Napkin clip							
Napkins							
Periodontal probe							
Pliers							
Polisher							
Resin							
Retractor							
Rongeur							
Rubber dam							
Rubber dam clamp							
Rubber dam frame							
Rubber dam punch							
Safety goggles (patient)							
Sealant							
Spatula							
Toothbrush							
Toothpaste							
Tray							
Wax							

Total for page _____

Notes

Medical Expenses

Physical Medicine

Item	Vendor	Price	No	Total	1	2	3
Activator							
Acupuncture needles							
Balance trainer							
Biofeedback							
Cold laser							
Compression garment							
Cupping set							
Diathermy							
Ear seeds							
Electrotherapy							
Exercise ball							
Exercise machine							
Exercise mat							
Foam roller							
Iontophoresis							
Joint supports							
Massage oil							
Massage roll							
Massage stones							
Massager							
Moxa							
Muscle stimulator							
Paraffin							
Pinch guage							
Resistance bands and tubing							
Skinfold calipers							
TENS unit							
Weights							

Tables

Item	Vendor	Price	No	Total	1	2	3
Adjustment							
Inversion							
Massage							
Massage chair							
Ob/Gyn							
Orthopedic							
Physical therapy							
Tilt							
Traction							
Weight bench							

Total for page _____

Notes

Extra Clothing

Keep an extra pair of clothes at work just in case.

Belt		Blouse	
Earrings		Eyewear	
Pants		Pantyhose	
Shirt		Shoes	
Skirt		Socks	
Undershirt		Underwear	

Extra Toiletries

Keep an extra pair of toiletries at work just in case. Avoid products with strong smells that may bother patients.

Item	Vendor	Price	No	Total	1	2	3
Blush							
Breath mints							
Chewing gum							
Contact solution							
Contacts							
Dental floss							
Deodorant							
Ear swabs							
Eyeliner							
Foundation							
Fingernail file							
Hair dryer							
Hair gel or spray							
Hair razor (electric)							
Lip gloss							
Lipstick							
Lotion							
Mascara							
Nail clippers							
Nail file							
Nail polish							
Nail polish remover							
Powder							
Toothbrush							
Toothpaste							

Total for page _____

Notes

Chinese Herbs

Item	Vendor	Price	No	Total	1	2	3
Agastache							
Alangium							
Anemone							
Anisodus							
Ardisia							
Aster							
Astragalus							
Cannabis							
Carthamus							
Cinnamomum							
Cissampelos							
Coptis							
Corydalis							
Croton							
Daphne							
Datura							
Dendrobium							
Dichroa							
Ephedra							
Eucommia							
Euphorbia							
Flueggea							
Forsythia							
Gentiana							
Gleditsia							
Glycyrrhiza							
Hydnocarpus							
Ilex							
Ligusticum							
Lobelia							
Phellodendron							
Platycladus							
Pseudolarix							
Psilopeganum							
Pueraria							
Rauwolfia							
Rehmannia							
Rheum							
Rhododendron							
Saussurea							
Schisandra							
Scutellaria							
Stemona							
Stephania							
Styphnolobium							
Trichosanthes							
Wikstroemia							

Source: Wikipedia

Total for page _____

Notes

Naturopathic Herbs

Item	Vendor	Price	No	Total	1	2	3
Alfalfa							
Ashwaganda							
Black cohosh							
Burdock							
Calendula							
Chamomile							
Chaste tree							
Coltsfoot							
Comfrey							
Cramp bark							
Dandelion							
Echinacea							
Elderberry							
Eleuthro							
Feverfew							
Ginger							
Ginkgo							
Goldenrod							
Gotu kola							
Hawthorne berry							
Holy basil							
Hops							
Kava							
Lemon balm							
Licorice (DGL)							
Milk thistle							
Motherwort							
Nettles (freeze dried)							
Oat seed							
Oregon grape root							
Pau d'arco							
Poke root							
Psyllium husk							
Red clover							
Sage							
Saw palmetto							
Slippery elm							
St. John's wort							
Thuja							
Turmeric (curcumin)							
Uva ursi							
Valerian root							
Wild yam							
Witch hazel							
Wormwood							
Yarrow							
Yellow dock							

Total for page _____

Notes

Supplements

Homeopathics

Item	Vendor	Price	No	Total	1	2	3
Aconitum							
Arsenicum							
Apis							
Arnica							
Aurum							
Belladonna							
Bryonia							
Calcarea carbonicum							
Causticum							
Ignatia							
Kalium carbonicum							
Lachesis							
Lycopodium							
Natrum muriaticum							
Nux vomica							
Phosphorus							
Phytolacca							
Pulsatilla							
Rhus toxicodendron							
Sepia							
Silicea							
Staphysagria							
Sulphur							
Veratrum alba							

Nutrients

Item	Vendor	Price	No	Total	1	2	3
5-HTP							
Acetyl L-carnitine							
Aloe vera							
Alpha lipoic acid							
Arginine							
Bioflavonoid							
Castor oil							
Coconut oil							
Coenzyme Q10							
Chondroitin							
Cranberry							
DHEA							
Digestive enzymes							
Fiber							
Fish oil (DHA/EPA)							
Flax seed (ground)							
GABA							
Garlic							

Total for page _____

Notes

Nutrients (continued)

Item	Vendor	Price	No	Total	1	2	3
Glucosamine							
Glutamine							
Glycine							
Grapefruit seed extract							
Lysine							
Mannose							
Melatonin							
MSM							
Pregnenolone							
Probiotics							
Progesterone							
Protein powders							
Quercitin							
Red yeast rice							
Resveratrol							
Taurine							
Tyrosine							

Formulas

Item	Vendor	Price	No	Total	1	2	3
Adrenal							
Allergy							
Antibacterial							
Antiviral							
Anti-inflammatory							
Cardiovascular							
Detox							
Eyecare							
Gallbladder							
Gastrointestinal							
Glucose regulation							
Immune system							
Kidney							
Liver							
Men's health							
Mind and focus							
Musculoskeletal							
Neural							
Respiratory							
Sleep aid							
Sinus							
Thyroid							
Urinary							
Women's health							

Total for page _____

Notes

Supplements

Minerals

Item	Vendor	Price	No	Total	1	2	3
Betaine HCl							
Calcium							
Charcoal (poisonings)							
Chromium							
Iron							
Magnesium							
Potassium							
Selenium							
Trace minerals							
Zinc							

Vitamins

Item	Vendor	Price	No	Total	1	2	3
Retinoids (A)							
B complex							
Thiamine (B1)							
Riboflavin (B2)							
Niacin (B3)							
Pantothenic acid (B5)							
Pyridoxal phosphate (B6)							
Folate (B9)							
Methylcobalamin (B12)							
Ascorbic acid (C)							
Cholecalciferol (D)							
Tocopherol (E)							
Phylloquinone (K)							
Multivitamin							

Website list

Lucky Vitamin	luckyvitamin.com
Mountain Rose Herbs	mountainroseherbs.com
Rx Homeo	rxhomeo.com
Vitacost	vitacost.com

Total for page _____

Notes

Management Experience

Continuining education
SBA or SCORE training

☐

Mentoring or supervising
Work experience (associate position, residency)

☐

Professional Fees

Item	Vendor	Total
Certifications		
Continuing education		
CPR/AED certification		
DEA number		
Professional association (national, state)		
Professional license		
National Provider Identifier	https://nppes.cms.hhs.gov	**Free**

Remedy Books

Item	Total
Concepts in Health Care Entrepreneurship	
Concepts in Health Care Entrepreneurship: Summary Guide	
Go online to remedybooks.com and download learning materials	**Free**

Additional Expenses

Item	Vendor	Price	No	Total	1	2	3

Total for page _____

Notes

Miscellaneous

Additional Expenses

Item	Vendor	Price	No	Total	1	2	3

Total for page _____

Notes

Financing Sources

Personal Sources

Cancelling a permanent life insurance policy ☐

Permanent life insurance cash value loan ☐

Retirement plan withdrawal ☐

Income (self-employment, job) ☐

Retirement plan loan (401k, qualified plan) ☐

Savings ☐

Private Sources

Grants and venture capital are rare but search online, including local nonprofit websites, and contact a local SBA or SCORE office. Compile a proper loan agreement to avoid tax problems for the lender.

Cosigner or guarantor ☐

Friend ☐

Significant other ☐

Family member ☐

Grant ☐

Venture capital ☐

Commercial Loans

Cash flow loan (SBA 7a loan program) ☐

Line of credit (home equity) ☐

Collateralized loan (SBA 504 loan program) ☐

Mortgage equity withdrawal ☐

Financial institution	*APR*	*Financial institution*	*APR*
_____	_____	_____	_____
_____	_____	_____	_____
_____	_____	_____	_____

Loan procedure

Business plan with *résumé* ☐

Review credit reports and FICO score ☐

Personal financial statements ☐

Tax returns (last several years) ☐

Website list

CIT Small Business Lending	cit.com
GE Health Care Finance	gehealthcarefinance.com
Professional Practice Capital	ppcloan.com
Rx Financial Group	rxfinancialcorp.com
Wells Fargo Practice Finance	practicefinance.wellsfargo.com

Seller Financed Loan

Business valuation ☐

Escrow agent ☐

Succession plan ☐

Covenant not to compete ☐

Negotiation matrix ☐

Term life insurance ☐

Loan agreement terms

Amortization schedule ☐

Breach of contract (specify breaches) ☐

Down payment ☐

Maturity date ☐

Buyer default ☐

Collateral ☐

Interest rate (above IRS minimums) ☐

Principal-agent relationship ☐

Notes

Work through the business valuation project online at remedybooks.com. Activity related to a building or land should be excluded from a business valuation. Use Microsoft Excel to set up the cash flow projection.

Weighted Average Cost of Capital

1. Market rate of debt _____ x (1 – Applicable tax rate) _____ = _____ Modified rate of debt

2. Modified rate of debt _____ x Target percentage of debt _____ = _____ Debt component

3. Market rate of equity _____ x Target percentage of equity _____ = _____ Equity component

4. Debt component _____ + Equity component _____ = _____ WACC (discount rate)

Long-term economic growth rate (terminal year) _____

Revenue Forecast
Set up revenue assumptions and establish future cash flows for the next five years plus a terminal year.

Economic outlook (see *Economic Research*)	☐	Historical trends (use accrual financial statements)	☐
Specific activity	☐	Immediate decline in patients	☐
Continuing patients	☐	New patients	☐
Returning patients	☐	Patient margin	☐

Expense Forecast
Set up expense assumptions and establish future cash flows for the next five years plus a terminal year. Adjust amounts for future inflation rates. Fixed expenses may need to be allocated to revenue according to its source.

Fixed expenses (partial allocation, segmentation)	☐	Historical trends (use accrual financial statements)	☐
Specific activity	☐	Variable expenses (percentage of revenue)	☐

Free Cash Flow Adjustments

Free cash flow to the firm		*Free cash flow to equity*	
Add back interest expense to net profit	☐	Deduct taxes (tax accountant, CPA)	☐
Deduct taxes (tax accountant, CPA)	☐	Change in working capital	☐
Change in working capital	☐	Add back depreciation expense	☐
Add back depreciation expense	☐	Deduct equipment purchases (cash)	☐
Deduct equipment purchases (cash)	☐	Deduct loan payments	☐

Practice Loan

APR (financial institution)	_____	Principal (should not exceed business value)	_____
Number of periods (months)	_____	Tax rate (tax accountant)	_____

1. APR _____ x (1 – Applicable tax rate) _____ = _____ Modified APR

2. Insert the modified APR, number of periods, and principal into Microsoft Excel's =PMT function

3. Insert the WACC (*see above*), number of periods, and payment (*Step 2*) into Microsoft Excel's =PV function

Project Evaluation

Cash shortfalls	☐	Internal rate of return	☐
Net present value	☐	Payback period (discounted)	☐
Payback period (undiscounted)	☐	Ratio analysis	☐

Notes

Documents

Billing

Billing policy (have patients sign) ☐	Credit card receipt (staple to service receipt) ☐
Collection letter ☐	Form CMS-1500 ☐
Invoice with payment terms ☐	List of common ICD codes ☐
List of "red flag" codes ☐	Low-income assistance application ☐
Medicaid claim form ☐	Medicare claim form ☐
Missed appointment policy (have patients sign) ☐	Payment receipt ☐
Payment plan options ☐	Service receipt with patient's specific ICD codes ☐
Superbill with common ICD codes ☐	Worker's compensation claim form ☐

Employees

Be careful never to ask questions or discuss subject matter covered by employment laws when hiring employees.

Cash budget (see remedybooks.com) ☐	Employee handbook (employees sign) ☐
Form I-9, uscis.gov ☐	Form W-4, irs.gov ☐
IRS publications 15 and 15A ☐	Job listings ☐
Job procedures ☐	Offer letter (hiring a candidate) ☐
Patient privacy (employees sign) ☐	Safety posters, osha.gov ☐
Thank you letter (interview candidates) ☐	Worker protection posters, bls.gov ☐

Organization

Clinic overview and mission statement ☐	Fax cover sheet ☐
Health care provider biographies ☐	HIPAA compliance (third parties sign) ☐
Independent contractor work agreement ☐	Map and driving instructions to the clinic ☐
Map and driving instructions to labs or imaging ☐	Material safety data sheet ☐
OSHA Form 300, osha.gov ☐	Product catalogs ☐
Supplement order forms ☐	Vendor contracts ☐

Patient Care

Diet diary ☐	Education materials (brochures) ☐
Diagnostic imaging order forms ☐	General wellness guide ☐
Lab order forms ☐	List of referral recommendations (specialists) ☐
Meal plans (diabetes, anti-inflammatory) ☐	Refusal of service waiver ☐
Release of records ☐	Review of systems checklist ☐
Side effects and interactions (drug, supplement) ☐	Treatment plans ☐

Procedures Manual

Accident reporting ☐	Administrative duties ☐
Biohazard handling and cleanup ☐	Emergency responses (fire, injury) ☐
Inventory tracking ☐	Lab specimen handling ☐
Privacy protection (HIPAA compliance) ☐	Treatment protocals (nurse, alternate provider) ☐

Notes

Documents

Patient Chart
Include copies of billing and patient care documents when applicable.

Advanced directive	☐	Chart notes	☐
Consent forms (general and specific)	☐	Demographic census	☐
Intake forms (general and specific)	☐	Interoffice notes	☐
Lab results (pertinent findings)	☐	Lab tracking list (ordered labs)	☐
Mental health questionnaires	☐	Physical screening questionnaires	☐
Prescriptions tracking list (refills)	☐	Privacy waiver (insurance billing)	☐
Symptom assessment and tracking	☐	Visit expectations (patients fill out while waiting)	☐

Tax Documents

Bank statements	☐	Charge card statements	☐
Employee timecards	☐	Forms 1098 and 1099 from other entities	☐
Mileage log (personal vs. business use)	☐	Processed checks	☐
Receipts with business purpose written on back	☐	Vendor invoices	☐

Calendar Reminders

Antidiscrimination training	☐	Antiharassment training	☐
Connect with referral sources	☐	Connect with support network	☐
Corporate governance meeting (attorney)	☐	Employee reviews	☐
HIPAA compliance training	☐	Monthly staff meetings	☐
Review of clinic (retention checklist)	☐	Safety training (OSHA compliance)	☐

Calendar date	Reminder alert
January 1	Submit fourth estimated tax payment by January 15 (for prior year)
January 1	Send independent contractors Form 1099 before January 31
January 1	Issue employees Form W-2 before January 31
January 1	Submit Form 1096 to the IRS by January 31
March 1	Submit corporate tax forms or extension to IRS by March 15
April 1	Submit first estimated tax payment by April 15
April 1	Submit personal and other business tax returns or extensions to IRS by April 15
June 1	Submit second estimated tax payment by June 15
September 1	Submit third estimated tax payment by September 15
October 1	Order holiday cards
November 1	Mail holiday cards

Notes

Dear Reader,

I hope that this information improves your ability to succeed as a health care provider and form a smooth-running clinic that adds to your enjoyment of work and life.

I would appreciate your help letting other health care providers know about this clinic checklist. At your convenience, could you please email or post online a recommendation for this book along with a thought about what you learned?

You are always welcome to email me at **info@remedybooks.com** and list ways in which I can improve the content of this book. I also welcome questions meant to better understand the content of this book or simply work through business issues you are facing.

I worked tirelessly for 10 years with great sacrifice so that the health care community would have a powerful, inexpensive way to learn about business and I want nothing more than to see you flourish. I am open to helping you any way I can.

Best Regards,
Jenson Hagen

Made in the USA
Charleston, SC
12 February 2013